Secrets to Prevent or REVERSE Osteoporosis & Osteopenia

The Natural - Drugfree Way -
with Simple Nutritional Changes and Exercise

by **Muryal Braun**

About The Author

Muryal is passionate about good nutrition since she nearly died at the age of 39, due to peritonitis. She had developed an internal abscess following surgery, that broke (during the surgical removal two years later), spreading the staphylococcus infection throughout her body.

Shortly before entering the hospital for that surgery, a fellow nurse casually handed her a copy of a book by Adele Davis, saying, "I don't know what you think about vitamins, but this is very interesting reading."

(Muryal had not taken any vitamins as her nursing professors had "pooh-poohed" them all through her training.)

However, after a lengthy hospital stay, she was so thin and weak that the surgeon told her it "might be a good idea to take some vitamins" if she had any at home. This caused her to think, "This is no coincidence."

Not having strength to do anything else when she got home, she began to read the book her friend had given her and it was so exciting she couldn't put it down. Until that point, her menu planning consisted of food that she thought was healthy, but mostly it was whatever tasted good, was quick to prepare, inexpensive and that her husband and the kids enjoyed eating.

Her entire life was changed from that time on. She read case studies all through the book about patients that doctors in the Los Angeles, CA area had referred to Nutritionist, Adele Davis because they didn't respond to conventional medical treatment for illness. It was fascinating reading, and she began to change the way she thought about food immediately.

By applying the principles in this book to her own life, and because of God's blessing, she has been able to enjoy abundant health and total healing from two hip fractures and two subse - quent surgeries to remove the hardware each time.

Muryal has said, "I can't tell you how much I appreciate my family putting up with my food experiments until I figured out how to make recipes healthier – but still tasty".

Her grown kids still talk about the time that she told them she was making "Orange Popsicles". The recipe called for freezing yogurt mixed with equal amounts of frozen concentrated orange juice. Sadly, any similarity between the outcome and orange popsicles was in name only.

Another time she tried "Blonde Brownies" using black strap molasses and whole wheat flour. Yuk!! Of course, they were not at all like yummy chocolate brownies, so it was a double whammy for her kids to have told them what she was making.

Needless to say, she totally backed away from any new food experiments for a while and then just sneaked good things in gradually, in small amounts without telling anyone, and to her amazement, it worked! The family got over being suspicious of everything she made and enjoyed meals again.

Muryal's discoveries really paid off years later, when she had two painful accidents that resulted in breaking the same hip TWICE. person be?). The first time, the doctor thought it was due to osteoporosis. So she researched everything she could find about bone health and applied everything she learned.

And guess what her surgeon said after the second accident? He explained that the reason it had broken the second time was not due to osteoporosis where the bone is weak and porous but because of the angle of the fall. He told her that when he "drilled through the bone where it had previously been broken, it was as hard as hard wood." See Doctor's Surgical Report at end of this book   He was extremely pleased with how fast it healed. And it is still very strong today—20years later!

She hesitated when it was suggested that she write this book, but became more than willing when so many friends and relatives told her they had been diagnosed with osteopenia or osteoporosis.

Because they were being urged to take useless, dangerous drugs, Muryal realized the need to share the "secrets" she had accumulated through the years to help prevent pain for others. <u>She uses the words "secrets" in her title because these truths are so often willfully hidden from the general public.</u>

She is grateful to her daughter, Carla, who for years encouraged her to share her nutritional research and also to her son, Dan, who helped with the editing.

Muryal says she has been enriched by so many integrative doctors (who use both alternative and traditional medicine), and researchers that it would be impossible to name them all.

Her prayer for you is that you may be blessed with abundant health.

Table of Contents

PART III: Secret Programs that Prevent and Reverse Osteopenia and Osteoporosis

INTRODUCTION

I decided to rewrite this introduction when my doctor urged me many times to have a Dexa Bone Density Scan after I broke my shoulder in 2010. It occurred to me that this is the starting point and may have been what brought you to this book, because that is where the diagnosis of osteopenia or osteoporosis usually begins.

After a bone density test, the next step is for the doctor to recommend a bone density drug, and it goes down hill from there.

(Chapter 9 of this book has more on drug dangers.)

Is The Dexa Bone Density Scan A Scam?

In the fall of 2010, while out for a two mile speed

walk with my daughter, I tripped and took a nose dive onto cement, landing hard on my right arm and shoulder. The impact caused severe bruising and broke my shoulder. When the orthopedic surgeon told me I might need surgery to "pin" my shoulder, I decided to apply what I had learned about bones and nutrition to this situation. He was stunned at my follow-up visit just four weeks later. The x-rays that were taken showed I was two weeks ahead of schedule in the healing process and I would definitely not need surgery!

After my shoulder healed, my primary doctor recommended that I have a Dexa Bone Scan, without even asking about the circumstances of my fall! (A tell-tale sign of osteoporosis is a broken bone occurring during a minor fall.) He said that he advised all patients over 65 who fall and break a bone to have one. From his training, he believed it was the best way to see if I had osteoporosis. I was convinced I did not have osteoporosis because my shoulder had healed so quickly.   I do not like to have any type of radiation that is not absolutely necessary, so I checked out all the information I had accumulated on Dexa Scans. My research has shown me that this scan is not all it's cracked up to be.

In an article by Dr. Nan Fuchs in her Women's Health Letter, November 2009, she warned that the most often used, "**DEXA Bone Density Test is not reliable for determining if a person has osteopenia or osteoporosis**".

Many think of bones as just dry posts to give our bodies a frame to hang our flesh on. Instead, bones are living tissue that is constantly being renewed. As we age, our old bone tissue may break down faster than it is replaced. So our bones become gradually porous and more fragile. The word osteoporosis means "porous bones".

Please consider the following problems with

the DEXA Bone Density Scan:

1. The density of the bone is shown just for that day. It does not show if the bone is stronger or weaker than it was before.

2. If you have had only one scan, and have been diagnosed with osteopenia or osteoporosis, it means your bones have been compared with a healthy 30 year old as normal. As every body is different, it is easy to see that a diagnosis based on this criteria could certainly be flawed.

3. You must wait a year or two for another test to compare with your first one to get a more accurate personal assessment.

4. When the next test is done, if the technician does not aim the X-ray at exactly the same spot on the same bone as the previous test, the test will not be dependable. If it is off by only 1/16th of an inch the results could be different from the previous scan, even if the bone density has not changed.

5. The DEXA test cannot tell you how quickly your

bones are breaking down.

Dr. Fuchs recommended a more reliable check for bone density that can tell you how well the re-modeling is working and how quickly you are losing bone. It is a simple urine test called Pyrilinks-D.

When bone breaks down it produces something called Dpd which is excreted in your urine. The Pyrilinks-D test measures the Dpd in your urine and tells you if your bones are breaking down faster than they're being rebuilt. The test can be performed every few months for comparison, and it is covered by most insurance companies. There are several labs that do the test now, so be sure to ask your doctor if you can have this test done instead of the DEXA test. The Pyrilinks-D test will give you immediate results.

Another problem with the Bone Density Scan is that:

Bone Density does not always equal Bone Strength.

On the well respected medical website Webmd.com, we read, "If your bone density is lower than normal, you can take steps to increase your bone strength and reduce your chances of having a fracture…"

This statement implies that by increasing your bone density you are also increasing your bone strength.

Unfortunately, that is not always true, as many have learned the hard way. If you have taken a bone density drug, you may have increased your "apparent" bone mineral density (BMD) while actually reducing the strength of your bones.

How could your bones become weaker after taking a "bone density drug"?

It can only be explained if you examine the process

by which the bisphosphonate drugs, such as Fosamax, Boniva, Actonel, Zometa, Aredia and the generic ones, seem to increase bone density. To keep our bones strong, there is a normal process of constant remodeling.

When you remodel a room of your house, you remove the old structure or fixtures and replace them with something newer or better. Bones are remodeled as the old bone cells (called osteoclasts) take calcium out of the bones. Those cells are then replaced by new bone cells (called osteoblasts) which bring fresh calcium and other minerals into the bones.

All of the bisphosphonate drugs prevent the osteoclasts from removing your old bone cells. This makes the bones look denser which gives you a false sense of security. But recent findings have proved that the **result is not stronger bones.**

Rather, the "denser bones" which have an increased amount of old bone tissue are more brittle and therefore break more easily than normal bones.

An increasing number of women have had the painful experience of having what is called an "atypical thigh bone fracture". While walking along casually they suddenly had a thigh bone break in a strange way.

There have been enough cases of these "atypical thigh fractures" in women who have been taking Fosamax, Boniva and other bisphosphonate drugs to cause the FDA to issue a statement of warning, acknowledging the connection.

If your doctor encourages you to have a Bone Scan, please request the preferred Pyrilinks-D test instead. And if it reveals that you are losing bone tissue faster than it is being replaced, why not talk to your doctor about using Strontium Citrate instead of drugs? That mineral has been shown in many studies and in actual patient tests to cause the bones to become stronger – not just "denser" looking.

Some doctors still recommend the Dexa Test because they believe the insurance companies will not pay for the newer test, but now most of them will. My primary doctor told me this when I broke my shoulder. He also said that he recommends the bisphosphonate drugs because <u>Medicare requires him to do so.</u>

I can't help questioning why Medicare requires it.

The following headline appeared in the news on 03/08/2010 referencing the bisphosphonate drugs: "Osteoporosis Drug Blamed for Leg Breaks". And the subheading..."Commonly prescribed drug meant to strengthen bones may have the opposite effect".

After another six months, on 10/13/2010, the FDA finally issued a requirement for the pharmaceutical companies to put a warning on the label of the bisphosphonates stating that they "may cause thigh fractures". I believe it is sad when one branch of our government requires something that another branch has warned against.

[10-13-2010] "The U.S. Food and Drug Administration (FDA) is updating the public regarding information previously communicated describing the risk of atypical fractures of the thigh, known as subtrochanteric and diaphyseal femur fractures, in patients who take bisphosphonates for osteoporosis. This information will be added to the Warnings and Precautions section of the labels of all bisphosphonate drugs approved for the prevention or treatment of osteoporosis.

Although it is not clear if bisphosphonates are the cause, these unusual femur fractures have been predominantly reported in patients taking bisphosphonates.

The bisphosphonates affected by this notice are only those approved to treat osteoporosis, including Fosamax, Fosamax Plus D, Actonel, Actonel with Calcium, Boniva, Atelvia, and Reclast *(and their generic products)."*

FDA.gov/newsevents/Newsroom/pressannouncements/ 2010/ucm229171.htm

Since we are the ones who must live with the consequences of decisions made concerning our health, we must be involved in that process, or the treatment may have a far worse impact on our lives than the illness.

The only way to truly increase bone density and make your bones stronger is by changing your lifestyle. This must include a healthy diet, a few supplements to provide the vitamins and minerals your bones need and some simple exercises.

It is my hope that you can avoid many of the problems that I faced and walk, or run, for as many years as you desire. Be assured of this truth: I am living proof that you can re-grow strong, healthy bone even after 65 years of age. This means you can reverse osteopenia and osteoporosis or avoid them entirely without using dangerous drugs if you will apply the findings in this book. The medical community may still state that it is impossible to naturally reverse osteoporosis, but now you can know there is hope and help for you.

PART ONE

Secret Minerals

that Prevent or Reverse

Osteopenia and

Osteoporosis

Chapter One

Calcium

How Can the Right Amount Leave Me Lacking?

Are you one of approximately 60 million Americans who experience heart burn and think you're getting your calcium from your antacid tablet?

Calcium is necessary for healthy bones, muscles, nerves, eyes and other tissue. (Remember, your heart is your biggest muscle.)

However, many are unaware of other factors that play a significant role in the body's use of calcium.

Because of all the "Drink Milk " commercials and other misinformation in the media, many people are convinced that drinking milk and eating other dairy products (even ice cream) will produce healthy bones and teeth. Sadly, that is not true.   Calcium alone is not the answer. Without adding other necessary nutrients and taking away some of the non-foods we are eating, calcium cannot be used by your body.

Even though a person may be sure that they are getting enough sources of calcium in their diet and may even be taking calcium supplements, the reasons why calcium may not be usable by the body have remained largely "secrets" because they have not been revealed to the public.

Secret Factors That Play a Role in the Body's Use of Calcium

The digestive process is a fascinating journey. Two major factors cause your food to be used more efficiently. The first is good initial chewing. The second is the availability of the proper acids. Our mouths and stomachs produce digestive juices to help break our food down thoroughly. The more completely it is broken down, the more readily the body can use it. And guess why that's so important? Because even if it's broken down well, much of the calcium you ingest may still be eliminated without being used by your body.

It is a well known fact that calcium supplements are often wasted. In some hospitals, calcium tablets are called "bedpan bullets" by the hospital staff because they are expelled completely undigested.

And here's why...

In order for calcium to be digested properly, the stomach needs to be acidic. In other words, our bodies need hydrochloric acid in the stomach for proper digestion. However, when we eat lots of starchy or sugary foods that neutralize the acids, causing digestive problems, many are convinced that they need to swallow antacids... you may even have some in your medicine cabinet, pocket or purse right now. Please throw them out!!

The problem is that these products neutralize the hydrochloric acid, so the food cannot be digested properly and is just pushed through the stomach in an undigested state. So instead of causing better digestion, antacids cause poor digestion and, with time, unhealthy bones and bodies. That is only one of the reasons to avoid using antacids.

Here's where it gets even more exciting. Many

alternative doctors agree that particularly after the age of 50, most people do not produce enough hydrochloric acid, which means that their food already cannot digest properly. Instead, it just rots in the stomach and produces lactic acid. It is this lactic acid (not hydrochloric acid) that makes people uncomfortable, causing "acid indigestion".

By increasing their hydrochloric acid, many people over fifty, have not only cured their digestive problems, but have also allowed their bodies to effectively use the minerals in their food for stronger bones and better health in general!

Are you one of the parents who get their children to drink milk by offering chocolate milk or a dessert with it? Chocolate milk has benefits, as cocoa contains needed magnesium, and milk contains protein. However, the sugar or other sweetener in the milk, causes an alkaline condition in the intestines that prevents the minerals from being used by your body. If your children have become addicted to chocolate milk, please replace the sugar or aspartame with the all natural sweeteners-- stevia, xylitol or erythritol. (Please note that honey has the same alkalizing effect as sugar in the digestive tract. I do recommend honey in preference to table sugar because it has some nutritive value but it should be used sparingly.)

Many years ago, I had a friend who said she did not like milk, so she never drank it unless she had chocolate cake to go with it.   After I became aware of these secret calcium factors, I began to wonder how many of us are increasing our chances of getting osteopenia or osteoporosis by combining our milk with sugar or starchy foods.

Major Food Sources:

Some foods that are high in calcium are dairy foods (particularly milk, yogurt, cottage cheese and hard unprocessed cheese); calcium-enriched orange juice, molasses, and rice beverages.

I no longer recommend soy products due to the fact that most soy farms now use genetically modified seeds which are called GMO. If you use soy please make sure it is GMO free.

Chapter 2

Magnesium

Is The Secret 50/50 Factor Working For You?

Magnesium is the fourth most abundant mineral found in the body. And about 50% of the body's total magnesium resides in the bones. A magnesium deficiency affects the hormone which helps regulate calcium.

Magnesium is found in dark green leafy vegetables, but how many of us eat enough of those? When you do, make sure they are as fresh as possible and the darker the better! If you prefer iceberg lettuce, for instance, you might get your family to eat higher nutrient greens by adding small pieces of darker greens and slowly increasing the amount.

Another source of magnesium is wheat bran, but this tends to be even more lacking in the American diet - without people even being aware of it! And the reason may surprise you. Many times I have heard friends say, "I always buy Wheat Bread." They often think they're getting a whole grain product just because they see "Wheat Bread" on the label.

Unfortunately, bread is able to be labeled "Wheat Bread" as long as the flour used comes from wheat. Note that many alterations can then occur that are NOT for the benefit of your health. "Wheat Bread" can often be composed mostly of bleached white flour which is always refined and processed which removes the magnesium-rich wheat germ and bran. In her book, <u>Eat Right to Keep Fit,</u> Adele Davis, states that after the vitamins are all removed from the wheat during the refining process, the commercial bakery often adds a few back and labels the bread as "enriched". She asked, "If someone robbed you of $100.00 and then gave you back $20.00 would you consider yourself enriched?" By removing the outer shell of the grain (which is called bran) and the germ in the center, the flour has no ingredients that will spoil. Now who profits from that? Definitely not you!

Not only have the vitamins been stripped away, but something has been added, BLEACH. Yup, the same stuff you use for your laundry! And you do know that chlorine bleach is a poison, right? So why would poison be added? You may like the first reason: it is added to make it whiter. Now here's the second reason: it provides an incredibly long shelf life for the product. Not only is it found in many packaged goods, but some don't even bear an expiration date because it can be stored indefinitely.

So, remember not to judge the quality of the bread by a browner color. Coloring has often been added to make it look darker like whole wheat. Unless you see the label "Whole Wheat" or "Whole Grain", it does not have the good, unadulterated flour in the product.

If you buy your bread, make sure the first ingredient is <u>whole wheat flour</u> and not just <u>wheat flour</u>. Wheat flour listed as the ingredient is unbleached or bleached flour.

So how can you protect yourself in home baking? You can immediately stop using bleached flour and substitute "Unbleached Flour" for the flour in your recipes. Unbleached flour does not have chlorine added to sky-rocket shelf life. Instead, it has a nice, creamy, natural color. You will see no difference in the looks, taste or texture of recipes.

• To take it to a higher level, though, wherever

possible try to use some 100% whole wheat flour along with unbleached flour in the recipe because it has so many added benefits. Start by substituting

whole wheat flour in small amounts and gradually increase by a tablespoon or quarter cup so it doesn't alter the texture and taste. (The ratio depends on the type of food. For a loaf of bread, a quarter of the flour could immediately be whole wheat. For pastries or cookies, it is best to begin with whole wheat pastry flour, for a smoother texture.)

• Please note: whole wheat flour also has good oil in it. So, if you intend to store it for more than a couple months, it is best to store it in the refrigerator to avoid having it get rancid.

We have often heard that people do not need food supplements. However, studies are increasingly finding that due to soil depletion and other environmental factors, most people now need added supplementation – especially for magnesium.

Dr.Michael R. Eades M.D. and his wife, Mary Dan Eades, M.D. state in their book, Protein Power, that if they had to recommend only one supplement, it would be magnesium because of its important role in so many bodily functions. When asked why it was not promoted more in the media, they replied that it is too inexpensive for the drug companies to promote so "it has no commercial lobby to tout its benefits on the airwaves."

Other Secrets That Play a Role in the Body's Use of Calcium

• Until recently, most nutritionists recommended only half as much magnesium as calcium. But, recent findings have shown that we need an equal amount of each.

• Dr. Nan Fuchs, in her Women's Health Letter, gave a vivid illustration that may help you understand this. Just what makes chalk different from ivory? Dr. Fuchs stated that chalk is a 100% calcium product. Then she explained that ivory is 50% calcium and 50% magnesium. Can you guess which one breaks easiest? You're right! While the chalk is very brittle and breaks easily, the ivory is almost unbreakable. Are your bones more like chalk or ivory? If you do not get enough magnesium, they are no doubt more like chalk.

Besides weak bones, a magnesium deficiency is also a common cause of hypertension (high blood pressure), heart attacks, abnormal heart rhythm, numbness, tingling, muscle cramps, constipation and seizures.

Major Food Sources :
Meats, green vegetables, avocados, seafood, potatoes, peanut butter, bananas, lima and kidney beans, peas, nuts, seeds, soy products, whole grains, dairy products and unsweetened cocoa powder.

Chapter 3

Phosphorus

Are You Overdosing On This One?

Ever heard a TV commercial telling you that phosphorus is important for strong bones?

Phosphorus is another necessary mineral for healthy bones.   In fact, eighty-five percent of your body's phosphorus is found in your bones. To be useful, however, it must not only be available to the body, but the amount must be <u>equal to the amount of calcium.</u>

Secret Factors That Play A Role in The Body's Use of Calcium

Bad sources of phosphorus that you DO eat can be as harmful to your bones as NOT eating good sources. In fact, one strongly-promoted dietary choice is causing devastating results today. The culprit is something that "fizzes" the calcium right out of you. Can you guess what it is? Few can believe that it's ... soft drinks! The reason is that soft drinks contain phosphoric acid, the part of the soda that gives it the fizz. And phosphoric acid is a derivative of phosphorous and too much of it produces an imbalance in your body.

Now how can you need phosphorus and yet not need it? Remember that your body needs it in EQUAL amounts to calcium. Too much phosphorus causes the body to pull calcium out of the bones in order to bring up the blood calcium level. Bone spurs and arthritis are caused when that old calcium is deposited in the joints. You might think, "If bone spurs and arthritis are caused by calcium deposits, it must mean the body has too much calcium. Right?"

Wrong! In fact, the opposite is true.
Instead of your body having too much calcium, your body may have too much phosphorus. And it can easily happen because phosphorous is not only prevalent in foods, but soft drinks are taking the place of a meal and even replacing water for many. Sadly, soft drinks have become a mainstay in our American diet.

Major Food Sources:

Nuts, seeds (sesame, sunflower,etc), dairy products, lentils, beans, peas, fish (especially sardines), other seafoods, meats, poultry, wheat germ and whole grains.

Chapter4

Strontium

The Little Known Mineral

Recent research has revealed some exciting news about this mineral, so I have added this chapter.

The fact that we need strontium for bones may be a new idea for you (as it was for me). So, what is strontium? It is a mineral closely related to calcium. We ideally have 350-400 milligrams in our bones and cartilage. The latest research using added strontium for bones has been very impressive.

A close friend of mine has battled cancer for several

years. First it was breast cancer. Then after surgery, chemo and radiation, it eventually metastasized to her bones. She recently had a break in her shoulder with no apparent cause. So this new research was very exciting for me to read and for her to hear.

After seeing such positive results for osteoporosis, others have gone on to study its effect for metastatic bone cancer.

The studies have proven that strontium...

• Provides protection for osteoporosis patients against fractures

• Causes improvement in osteoporosis quickly,   by stimulating new bone growth...

• Is so effective in replacing lost bone tissue that it even helps bone cancer patients grow new bone tissue...

So do we need strontium for bones? The latest research definitely says, "Yes."

Since this book mainly deals with osteoporosis and osteopenia, we'll consider that area first. One study was done with 353 women who had all suffered at least one fractured vertebrae due to osteoporosis.

Half the group took a patented strontium ranelate medication of 380 milligrams per day and the rest took a placebo. After one year, the group who took the strontium had a 3% increase in lumbar bone density. (However, strontium ranelate does have some serious side effect that the natural strontium does not have.)

At the end of the three year study, <u>the group that took the strontium had a 41 percent decrease in vertebral fractures, and an increase in their bone density by 11.4 percent</u> while the placebo group had a 1.3 percent decrease in their bone density.

The exciting news for my friend was another study done by Dr. Skoryna of McGill University in Montreal with metastatic bone cancer (a condition where cancer cells are multiplying out of control and slowly replacing bone tissue).   There was no known help for that problem until Dr. Skoryna experimented with only 272 mg/day of strontium gluconate for 3 months. (He used a lower dose for the strontium gluconate as he knew that strontium gluconate is absorbed much easier than the strontium ranelate.)

He discovered that with the strontium, new bone tissue grew to fill in some of the areas that had been eroded by the cancer. His <u>patients had a 172% increase in the rate of bone formation in just six months.</u> And these deposits were still visible on x-rays six months after the strontium had been discontinued!   Many of the cancer patients also experienced improved feelings of well being and even gained weight during the strontium experiments.

Some integrative doctors are now prescribing strontium in the form of strontium citrate for their osteoporosis patients because that is the form most easily absorbed. The recommended dose that they are using is 681 milligrams (3 capsules of 227 mg. each) at bedtime on an empty stomach or at least 2 hours after last meal and before next meal.

You should never take any calcium food or supplement at the same time as strontium or the strontium will be ineffective. The two minerals cannot be taken at the same time as the calcium is one step up on the mineral scale and as both compete for the same protein to carry them into the bone tissue, the calcium always wins.

Conclusion

Recapping, we have seen that if you want to grow healthy bones or if you want to reverse osteoporosis or osteopenia, you need equal amounts of calcium, magnesium and phosphorus.

Calcium is not enough!

Another very important factor, as we have mentioned, is that your stomach needs to have an acid condition to digest minerals properly. If sugary foods are eaten at the same time we consume calcium, the digestive system becomes alkaline and the calcium cannot be digested. Likewise, if you take an antacid (such as Tums or Tagamet) after a meal, it is impossible for your body to digest or benefit from the calcium in your diet or in the calcium-fortified Tums tablet.

By the way, are you aware that eating any white starchy foods, such as white flour or white rice, causes the same problem as eating sugary foods? This is because foods like white bread or bagels, potato chips, pretzels, white rice, white flour and spaghetti are converted into a simple sugar almost as soon as they are eaten.

But there's hope! Even though certain foods can prevent the absorption of calcium, just small changes in the way you eat can begin to restore health and reverse your bone loss.

PART TWO

Secret Vitamins

That Prevent or Reverse

Osteopenia and

Osteoporosis

Chapter 5

Vitamin D₃

Is Your Sunscreen Blocking it?

Secrets Concerning

Vitamin D's Role In the Body's Use of Calcium

Vitamin D is a fat-soluble vitamin that is rarely present in foods. But our bodies were designed so that when ultraviolet rays from the sun touch our skin, they trigger synthesis of this very necessary vitamin.

Vitamin D has many important functions. With respect to bone health, Vitamin D regulates both the calcium and phosphorous levels in the blood by enabling their absorption from food. Even though we may have enough acid in the stomach to break down the calcium in food for digestion, our bodies are unable to absorb calcium from our food into the blood stream without enough Vitamin D. And if calcium is not in the bloodstream, it cannot get to our bones.

It promotes bone growth and health, so a deficiency of Vitamin D can lead to bone softening. Known for preventing rickets in children it also works with calcium to protect older people from osteoporosis. Without Vitamin D, bones can become brittle, porous, thin and misshapen.

Have you seen any bow-legged children recently? Even some who have been drinking Vitamin D-

fortified milk?   Bow-leggedness is a symptom of
rickets which is caused by a deficiency of Vitamin D!
How can this be? The answer comes from what
seems to be a secret: There is more than one form
of Vitamin D.

The major forms of this fat soluable vitamin are
Vitamin D2 (or synthetic Vitamin D) and Vitamin D3
(the natural form). Vitamin D3 is produced in skin
exposed to sunlight, specifically ultraviolet B
radiation. It is significant to know that ONLY natural
Vitamin D3 can be absorbed and used by the body.

So, how do we get this natural Vitamin D3? Spend
at least 15-30 minutes in the sun each day <u>without
sunscreen.</u>

There is an irony here, though. Since just being
outside in the sun is a way to get Vitamin D3, we
should easily be able to get plenty of it.   But, again,

several "secret" factors can prevent that.

First: Since the invention of sunscreen, many are seriously lacking in Vitamin D because it can only be produced in your body through the interaction of the sun on cholesterol in your skin.   And sunscreen prevents the sun from working on any cholesterol you may have in your skin.

Second: If you have been using cholesterol lowering medications, they may have lowered your cholesterol to the point that the Vitamin D3 cannot be produced in the skin. (A dangerously low cholesterol level would be 100 to 150.)

Third: An often neglected fact about Vitamin D from sunshine is that the action of the sun on the cholesterol in the skin needs to be continued for 30 minutes or more after exposure, before washing the skin with soap to get optimal Vitamin D3 produced.

So as kind as you may think you are being to shower immediately, try postponing that shower if possible, or just use soap on the areas of the skin that have not been exposed to the sun.

Of course, it is best to avoid the sun in the hottest time of the day as well as overexposure. (Hottest hours are generally considered from noon to 3 p.m.) And it is better to have two shorter exposures than one long one.

Because of this lack of Vitamin D3 production, there's an additional loss: your bones will be unable to use calcium. And this all factors into arthritis as well.

Are you or your children drinking fat-free milk? There are two problems with fat-free milk: the lack of fat and the lack of Vitamin D3.   Another little known secret is that Vitamin D can only be absorbed in the presence of fat so you NEED good fats in moderation, such as butter, cream, olive oil or coconut oil in your diet for healthy Vitamin D absorption. A further reason why the Vitamin D in the milk is not usable by the body is because the form used is the synthetic Vitamin D2.

In talking with people of my "older" generation, it is interesting to note that it was very rare for a child to have a broken bone when we were young. In the summer, we spent most of our days outside in the sun, and a surprising amount of us were given one terrible tasting tablespoonful of Cod Liver Oil daily during the winter months. My mother always said, "Cod Liver Oil is cheaper than doctor bills", so we had to take it even during the depression.

Today, it is possible to get lemon flavored Cod Liver Oil and, anyone who has been diagnosed with osteopenia or osteoporosis will definitely be helped by taking 1 tablespoon Cod Liver Oil daily, or an even more potent krill oil which comes in a tiny capsule.

Think about it, former generations spent much of their time out of doors so they were able to get lots of sunshine to produce natural Vitamin D. And they did not have cholesterol lowering drugs or sunscreen. As Vitamin D has recently been proven to prevent infections and chronic illnesses, it is logical that a lack of this natural Vitamin contributes to the high incidence of cancer and heart disease as well as poor bone health.

Major Food Sources:

Vitamin D is rarely found in foods. As we have mentioned, it is almost impossible to get enough Vitamin D from our food supply. Even though Vitamin D is listed on the label of many foods, it is the synthetic form of the vitamin which does no good for your body. It is possible to get some of this natural vitamin in oily fish such as sardines or salmon. But the best source is still sunlight.

Chapter 6

Vitamin C

Do You Have Enough of the "Glue" that Retains Your Calcium?

Vitamin C is a water-soluble vitamin, meaning that what is not needed by the body is eliminated rather than stored, so there is never any danger of getting too much.

Is your first thought when you think of Vitamin C, "Oh, yes, the cold vitamin?" Or are you thinking, "I get plenty of that. I drink orange juice every day."

There has been much publicity concerning Vitamin C and the fact that it has been proven to prevent colds. But we seldom hear about the many other functions that Vitamin C has in our bodies. Much research has been done to show its importance for the entire immune system.

Three-time Nobel Prize Winner, Dr. Linus Pauling, for example, told of the importance of Vitamin C in fighting cancer in his book, *Cancer and Vitamin C.* In addition, the Cancer Centers of America have just recently been granted approval by the FDA to do some double-blind studies using Vitamin C for their cancer patients. Recent research has proven that it is important for the heart and nearly every cell in the body. However, the purpose of this chapter is to emphasize its part in growing healthy bones and in preventing or reversing osteopenia and osteoporosis.

Now for some trivia about Vitamin C:

Do you know why British sailors were called "Limies"? In the 18th Century, on long ocean voyages, British sailors were dying in great numbers from scurvy until it was found that the deaths were prevented by having the sailors eat <u>limes</u> every day.

Then, in 1931 it was discovered that 50 mg. of Vitamin C per day would prevent large scale out-breaks of scurvy.   However, the <u>symptoms of scurvy are still seen frequently today</u> (but they are not called scurvy):

> Tiredness (now called Chronic Fatigue?)
>
> Weakness
>
> Irritability
>
> Aches and pains throughout the body (now called Fibromyalgia?)
>
> Slow healing
>
> Internal bleeding
>
> Bruising easily

Dental symptoms, such as bleeding or swollen gums

Weak bones (osteopenia or osteoporosis?)

How many people do you know who have any of those symptoms?

Because we see so many cases of the above symptoms, most alternative doctors believe that our government recommended RDA of 60 - 90 mg. is ridiculously low. <u>Are you aware that your dog or cat produces about 3000-4000 mg. of Vitamin C every day? The only creatures on our planet that</u> do not produce Vitamin C are humans, monkeys and guinea pigs.

A Secret Factor That Plays a Role in the Body's Use of Calcium

Something that makes Vitamin C especially important for healthy bones is the fact that it helps to produce collagen. <u>Collagen</u> is a substance needed by every cell that acts like glue, and this is why it's invaluable:

As we have discussed, Vitamin D helps transfer calcium from food in the digestive tract into the bloodstream. So if you have enough of the true Vitamin D, your blood carries calcium to your bone cells. However, if there is no collagen in the cells of the bones to hold the calcium where it is needed, the calcium will just pass right through and be eliminated from the body!

After researching this topic for many years, I have increased the amount of raw vegetables and fruits in my diet and added generous amounts of Vitamin C supplements. I believe that has been a great factor in helping me to regrow healthy bones as well as for my general good health. In the last chapter of this book, I will share the amounts of the various vitamins and minerals that I have found to be adequate and that I recommend as a minimum for healthy bones.

Even if a person is able to consume several servings of fruits and vegetables each day, most nutritionists recommend supplementing the diet with extra Vitamin C because it is needed by every cell in your body.

Researchers have found that the best way to tell if we are taking enough Vitamin C is to up the dose until we start to have diarrhea, or to what is called the "bowel tolerance level," and then cut back just a little for the perfect dose.

Major Food Sources:

Fruits: apples, all kinds of berries, lemons, oranges, grapefruit, kiwi, cantaloupe, honeydew, watermelon, and tomatoes.

Vegetables: asparagus, broccoli, cabbage, cauliflower, kale, potatoes, and spinach.

Chapter 7

Vitamin K2

Until recently not much had been written about Vitamin K2 for healthy bones. You may have heard about the need for Vitamin K in relation to hemophilia. I was familiar with that as a child because a friend of mine had hemophilia and needed Vitamin K to help his blood to clot so he wouldn't bleed to death when he got a cut.

Vitamin K is important for bone health because of its function of activating enzymes responsible for bone formation. But you must be sure that you are getting K2. The vitamin K that is listed on many packaged foods, is synthetic and does no good for your body.

For maximum bone health, and all its other benefits, many nutritionists now recommend that you get between 85 to 100 mcg. of Vitamin K2 daily. But be sure to consult your health care professional before adding this to your routine — especially if you are on a blood thinning medication.

Part Three

Habits That Help
Prevent or Reverse
Osteopenia and
Osteoporosis

Chapter 8

Exercise

Another Secret Factor for Strong Bones

It is no secret that exercise is important for maintaining health. Walking or other weight-bearing exercise is usually recommended to help strengthen the muscles and bones. However, in 2003, a new concept hit the market that has caused quality exercise to be not only a possibility, but a wonderful opportunity for those who are not able to walk and for those who are not able to exercise outside or at a gym.

With bestsellers Protein Power (Bantam Books 1996) and the Protein Power Plan (Warner 2000), Dr. Mary Dan Eades and Dr. Michael R. Eades had become known primarily for their work in treating overweight and the metabolic syndrome. They had advocated strength training in both books as a necessary component with diet for weight loss. In their recent book, The Slow Burn Fitness Revolution: The Slow Motion Exercise That Will Change Your Body in 30 Minutes a Week (Broadway Books, 2003), they used their long history of nutritional and metabolic expertise to collaborate with Fredrick Hahn, a strength-training expert who had spent over twenty years refining the techniques of slow-speed strength training.

The book combines medicine, exercise, science, and weight-training. It reveals the benefits of simple resistance exercises with weights that are done very slowly to improve not only muscles, but also the bones. They were able to explain how developing your muscles always stimulates your bones to become stronger.

Even though she was very active until she was 90, my mother became unable to carry even a heavy purse. This motivated me to start strength training at age 65, when my son bought me a pair of small dumbbells. He told me that most people lose strength in their upper body as they age. Although I had been using the weights for a few years, I didn't enjoy using them until I implemented these Slow Burn exercises shortly after the book was published in 2003.

No pain; no gain?

What convinced me to start applying this program was the high recommendation from Dr. Bruce West, a cardiologist practicing in Monterey, CA. Dr. West is a former Olympic athlete who had kept in shape by spending many hours each week at the gym. In September, 2003, Dr. West shared in his Health Alert magazine that he had stopped his old routines in favor of the Slow Burn exercises and had saved many hours each week to enjoy time with his family.

Like Dr. West, I have found that a wonderful advantage to these exercises is that they only take 20-30 minutes and they only need to be done <u>once or twice a week.</u> You work with light weights. The workouts are not difficult and the results are better than aerobics. I highly urge you to make it part of your fitness program. Less time and less work for better results. I call that a winning combination!

I also am a strong advocate of swimming. I swim thirty laps every day during the summer months in my pool and really enjoy it, as I like an exercise that doesn't cause me to sweat – especially on a hot day.

Many fitness centers now provide group swimming exercises for Physical Therapy. Patients are thrilled to see excellent, painless improvement for many conditions as the water allows exercise benefits without stress on the joints. For dense, healthy bones, I hope you will try to find an exercise that you really enjoy and do it regularly!

Chapter 9

Secrets About

The Foods We Eat

How close are you to winning the
"Walking Garbage Can" award?

No book on any health topic is complete without
discussing the foods we eat.   In our day, many are
concerned with counting calories and avoiding fat.
This is the kind of diet that has produced so much
chronic illness in our country.

So they ignore the need for eating quality food that will build strong bones, muscles, nerves and other tissue and eat "fat-free" items with no nutritional value. No amount of supplements will replace good wholesome food! Our goal for each day must be to eat delicious, nutritious **FOOD.**

Every cell in your body must have **protein**. It is absolutely necessary for healthy skin, muscles, nerves, heart (remember, your heart is your biggest muscle), and brain tissue--and for the immune system, which fights disease and preserves your health.

In fact, research suggests that <u>cancer cells are present in all of us,</u> but they will only become out of control in a body with a weakened immune system. And how does that occur? <u>IN BODIES THAT LACK PROTEIN.</u> It is protein that produces the killer white blood cells that fight any kind of infection.

70

Two of the most readable books on the importance of protein and the bad rap it has gotten are the Protein Power Life Plan , and Protein Power (already mentioned in the previous chapter on exercise). Both books by Dr. Michael R. Eades and Dr. Mary Dan Eades tell of thousands of readers who have written them to share dramatic health improvements after just a few weeks of increasing their protein intake as recommended in those books.

Ironically, the prevalent, heavily promoted low-fat, high carbohydrate diets have caused many to become overweight and chronically ill.   Be encouraged that those conditions may be reversed quickly by applying a few easy steps to improve your food choices.   Just taking baby steps will get you headed in the right direction!   YOU CAN DO IT!

In order to have optimum health, a simple plan is to

eat plenty of fresh fruits and vegetables and get at least 20 grams of complete protein for each meal for an average person of about 150 pounds. Of course, that amount needs to be adjusted proportionately for body size.

Another area that is often misunderstood, is what constitutes good quality protein. Complete protein is any food that includes all ten of the <u>essential amino acids</u> which are the building blocks of protein. Many foods contain only a few of these amino acids. The reason they are called essential is that our bodies are not able to produce those amino acids so they must be obtained through our food. A problem with package labels is that the amount of protein listed does not differentiate between complete (having all 10 essential amino acids) and incomplete protein.

If you eat crackers that show 3 grams of protein per serving on the box, this is incomplete protein. To make it complete you would need to add some hard unprocessed cheese or other complete proteins. Other incomplete proteins can be mixed together to create complete proteins. An example would be whole grain rice and beans. Another example of that would be to combine whole grain cereal with milk, or beans with cheese. These are called complementary proteins. But it is difficult to obtain enough of the essential amino acids in that way, which is one reason why many vegetarians have heart problems.

Meat protein is the best source of Vitamin B 12 which is very much needed for a healthy heart.

Below, I have compiled a list of foods that are complete protein, and I hope you will get some protein from this list in every meal.

Quantity	Food Source	Protein Gms.
4 oz.	Lean Meat, Fish, Poultry	18-20
1 oz (1" cube)	Hard Cheese (unprocessed)	7
1/2 cup	Cottage Cheese	14

One	Medium Egg	8
1 cup	Milk	8
1/3 cup	Skim Milk Powder	8
1/2 cup	Nuts	14-22
1/2 cup	Raw (untoasted) Wheat Germ	24
1 cup	Milk (raw or organic)	7
1 cup	Yogurt	
	(Plain – no sugar or thickener)	8
1/2 cup	Tofu (only if organic source)	9

Sources below are good if combined with some complete proteins from the list above:

1 cup	Cooked Kidney Beans	16
1 cup	Cooked Oatmeal	6
2 Tbsp.	Almonds	7
1 cup	Cooked Brown Rice	15
1 cup	Cooked Whole Wheat Spaghetti	7

Recent research has shown that those who eat

the most protein have the strongest bones. So please enjoy your proteins.

Another crucial need for healthy bones is good fats. Some nutritional experts are recommending that we get half of our calories for each meal from healthy fats, so that we will be able to digest our minerals and make our meals more satisfaction. Remember, fats have twice as many calories per gram as carbohydrates, so it doesn't take a lot of fat to consume that amount. But your meals will be much more satisfying. These good fats also make it possible for us to burn unwanted body fat and protect our hearts with omega 3's.

Some examples of healthy fats are extra virgin olive oil, organic coconut oil, butter, nuts and avocados. Ever since the 1980's we have seen no fat or low fat diets and products promoted. So many have gone to the extreme and tried to eliminate fat from their diets. The result has been an alarming increase in heart attacks, osteoporosis, cancer and obesity. No one can be healthy while eating a fat free diet. One of the results of avoiding fat has been eating more carbohydrate rich junk food in the futile attempt to satisfy hunger.

So please be sure to incorporate healthy fats in your meals and avoid all the unhealthy hydrogenated oils which are in almost every packaged food product. Hydrogenated oils extend shelf life because they cannot get rancid. The good fats nourish the cell walls of our bodies so that disease cannot enter the cell. Bad fats clog the blood and produce poor cell walls all through our bodies - causing inflammation and every type of illness. Learn to read labels if you do buy packaged products

Chapter 10

Supplements

Not "If", but how many?

In our day, an increasing number of integrative doctors are now encouraging their patients to take food supplements to make up for what is lacking in our Standard American Diet- (better known as SAD).

I have added supplements to my diet to protect my bones as well as my heart, brain and immune system. Using knowledge that it took me years to acquire, may save you from having a hip fracture. Of course, it can happen to anyone if the bone receives enough pressure from the angle of a fall. But, if you do have an accident that causes an hip fracture and surgery, wouldn't you like to hear your surgeon remark after the surgery to repair it, that "you don't have osteoporosis"?

After surgery for my second broken hip, my surgeon told me that I should continue doing whatever I had been doing that caused me to have such strong bones.

Below are the supplements that I take each day:

Vitamin C	5000 mg
Vitamin D3	5000 IU (International Units)
Calcium	1000 mg (Chelated)

Magnesium Citrate 1000 mg

Phosphorus none (most get enough from food)

Boron   3mg

Betaine Hydrochloride 325 mg After hi-protein meal

Strontium Citrate   340 mg Once per week

(Recommended dose for osteoporosis 680 mg/day)

To keep joints well lubricated I also take:

MSM	500 mg
Glucosamine Sulfate	500 mg
Krill Oil	1000 mg
or Omega 3 fish oil	1000 mg

Also, for general health:

A Quality Multiple Vitamin –

Vitamin E d'alpha tocceropherols 400 IU

Coenzyme Q10   100 mg

I have used Puritan's Pride Vitamins and also Swanson's Vitamins for many years and I highly recommend them for quality as well as economy.

These recommendations are based upon my research and what I have found provides me with very healthy bones. They have not been evaluated by the FDA. I encourage you to seek the best for your body, and to be sure to contact your healthcare provider for any medical advice.

"The Hushed-Up DANGERS and LIES About

Bone Density Drugs!"

Can Fosamax or Other Drugs Increase Bone Density in Osteopenia or Osteoporosis?

Osteopenia is the word used to describe loss of bone density and is thought to be a precursor to Osteoporosis. The term "Osteopenia" did not even exist until a little over a decade ago. It became popular in medical literature about the same time as the drug Fosamax entered the market.

Though you follow all the proactive healthy eating and exercise habits recommended here, you may still experience painful, destructive, and even lethal, consequences if you take "bone-density" drugs. Please use this information to make wise decisions for your health.

Osteopenia refers to Bone Mineral Density (BMD) that is lower than normal peak BMD but not low enough to be classified as osteoporosis. Bone mineral density is a measurement of the level of minerals in the bones, which shows how dense and strong they are. If your BMD is low compared to normal peak BMD, you are said to have osteopenia. Having osteopenia means there is a greater risk, that you may develop osteoporosis, as time passes, a state where your BMD is very low compared to "normal".

What causes Osteopenia?

Theoretically, the denser your bones are at about age 30, the longer it takes to develop osteopenia or osteoporosis. For the average person (hopefully not you), bones start becoming thinner as people grow older because existing bone cells are reabsorbed by the body faster than new bone is made. As this occurs, the bones lose minerals, heaviness (mass), and structure, making them weaker and increasing their risk of breaking. Everyone begins losing bone mass after they reach peak BMD at about 30 years of age—unless preventive measures are followed.

Some people who are diagnosed as having osteopenia may not have bone loss; they may just naturally have a lower bone density. Osteopenia may also be the result of a wide variety of other conditions, disease processes, treatments or medications.

"Osteoporosis is an advanced condition in which the bones have become increasingly porous, brittle, and subject to fracture, owing to loss of calcium and other mineral components, sometimes resulting in pain, decreased height, and skeletal deformities: common in older persons, primarily post-menopausal women, but also associated with long-

term steroid therapy and certain endocrine disorders."

Women are far more likely to develop osteopenia and osteoporosis than men. This is because women have a lower peak BMD and because the loss of bone mass speeds up as hormonal changes take place at the time of menopause. It has been found that prescribed estrogen sometimes seems to help increase bone density. However, synthetic estrogen (HRT) supplementation has also been linked to higher incidence of breast and ovarian cancer and heart disease.

Osteoporosis, literally means "porous bones," a condition of weak and brittle bones — so brittle that even mild stresses like bending over to tie shoes, lifting a vacuum cleaner or coughing can cause a fracture. In most cases, bones weaken when you have low levels of calcium, phosphorus and other minerals in your bones.

A common result of osteoporosis is fractures — most of them in the spine, hip or wrist. Although it's often thought of as a women's disease, osteoporosis also affects many men. And aside from people who have osteoporosis, many more have low bone density.

In fact, I have many young friends who have been told that they have osteopenia. As a result, they have been prescribed a medication that they have been instructed to take for the rest of their lives! The medicine is extremely expensive, really ineffective for increasing bone quality, and as they have yet to find all the side effects, it appears that the only one who will really profit from it is the drug company that produces it.

In 2006, for example, these bone-density drugs became the second most profitable prescribed and used drug category in the United States, netting $3.2 billion in sales for the manufacturers.

The medical establishment and media have touted Fosamax, and similar drugs in the category of bisphosphonates, as the answer to bone density problems. That is far from the truth. Their "answer" only creates far greater problems.

Particularly when it comes to drugs, whenever you hear a medical pronouncement in the news, it is wise to note the source. We must realize that when we hear about drug research in the news, the report usually comes from the company that is producing the drug, so the chances of pro-drug bias are extremely high. It has been reported recently, that the pharmaceutical companies often fail to report to the FDA the negative effects that they have discovered when testing their drugs.

And when it concerns your bones, there is a natural solution that is incredibly safer and cheaper, and the user doesn't experience counterproductive side effects. Instead, the inclusion of several bone enhancing minerals and vitamins results in the growth of dense, strong bones. How do I know?

It happened for me!

Dr. Nan Fuchs, in her special report, _Bone Health News,_ (May 2008) has warned about the results of the bone density scan, it <u>appears</u> that the bone has become more dense after a patient has been on Fosamax for a year or two. However, the truth is that it is not due to new bone growth. The drug simply prevents the old calcium from leaving the bone in the natural break down and replacement process, called remodelling, that our Designer planned. Therefore the bone looks denser but at the same time it is becoming more brittle. How could that possibly be called a desirable drug effect?

• Dr. Robert Jay Rowen in his September 2007 health

letter, *Second Opinion,* warned that people who have been on bone density drugs for some time have begun to experience necrosis (death) of the jaw bone. He told of one patient who came to him after taking Fosamax for 9 years. She woke up one morning with excruciating pain in her jaw. But that was only the beginning of her painful ordeal. She endured repeated surgeries (finally replacing part of her jaw with titanium). She also had to take antibiotics to fight the infections of the jaw and lost several teeth. Now she has permanent loss of sensation on one side of her face.

• One case would be bad enough, but there are hundreds of people who have had similar experiences. Many are presently involved in a lawsuit against Merck because the drug producer ignored the Food and Drug Administration's August 2004 request to add a warning label to the drug container.

I must also caution you to avoid any long term use of Prednisone as that also causes bone necrosis (death) – usually in the joints. One brave survivor of that very painful disease, has started a non-profit organization to help prevent others from suffering.

More recently, it has been documented that the bisphosphonate drugs have also caused many cases of esophageal cancer.

It's never too late, or too early, to change.

You can take steps to keep your bones strong and healthy throughout life, as well as avoid the debilitating side effects of drugs. That is why I wrote, <u>Secrets to Prevent or REVERSE Osteoporosis and Osteopenia.</u>

• Having broken the same hip TWICE—and then having the bone heal as hard as hard wood, I can attest to the fact that there is a safer, far more successful way to increase bone health: several natural nutrients and simple exercise. After the second break, my surgeon assured me that when he

had to drill through the area where the bone had broken before, it was so strong that it was like drilling through hard wood. With my first break, the doctor thought I had osteoporosis. That started my research that has continued to the present to find these safe natural ways to restore and preserve bones.

By incorporating a few nutrients and incorporate them into your diet along with some simple, quick exercises, you will be able to prevent or reverse bone problems. Save yourself from the misery caused by exorbitantly expensive and extremely dangerous bone density drugs. Avoid an expensive path to pain and debilitation through healthy eating and simple, quick exercises. There is a safe, natural way to prevent or reverse bone loss.

Often I am told, "It's great that you are so healthy at your age that you can live such an active life. I hope I will be as healthy as you are when I reach your age." That remark really disturbs me because it sounds as though people think it is just a matter of chance or that they are not responsible for how they choose to eat and live now. What we do today determines our health or lack of it for our future.

I pray you may believe that by trusting God and making wise choices, it is possible for you to live an abundant, healthy life.

May God Bless you,

Muryal

The Surgical Report from my Orthopedic Surgeon

(I have included only the part that described
the condition of my bone)

" ....At this point we reamed the lag screw and then I attached a three hole135" side plate . I let the tension off the leg and then used the compression screw to compress the fracture. The patient's bone was very tight , in fact, I did tap the bone because the quality of the bone was very dense and somewhat sclerotic most likely due to her good health and the previous fracture that she had in this area.

Because of the basilar neck nature of the fracture I then used the cannulated AO screw system and I placed a guide pin under fluoro control above the lag screw running from the lateral cortex of the greater trochanter into the head. I measured this at 70 mm and then drilled it and placed a 70 mm cannulated screw to control derotation.

At this point, we irrigated the wound and I placed the large Hemovac drain and closed the wound in layers with 1 vicryl pulling the vastus lateralis together, then the tensor fascia. I used interrupted sutures of 0 for the deep layer of the fat and then the subq. was closed with 2-0 vicryl. Once this was closed we then closed the skin with staples and the drain was sewn in,   A sterile dressing was applied and the patient was removed from the operating table and taken to the Recovery Room in a stable condition. C-arm x-rays of her hip in surgery looked very good. We are going to get permanent films. We are going to start her on physical therapy. I am going to check her clinical course over the next few days. I am giving her some coumadin for DVT and PE control and we are going to follow her along medically over the next few days."

D D : I 0 / 3 I / 92
D T : I I / 0 I / 9 2

Made in the USA
Middletown, DE
06 May 2024

53919501R00053